# Why you SHOULD NOT Exercise when you are dieting

**Theira Añez Ferrer**
**and**
**Delia Añez Ferrer**

# Index

# INTRODUCTION

To reach your desired weight and keep it with no effort, is that even possible? Well let me tell you that yes, it is possible, it's your decision; you are the only one that can make it happen. I did it… I still do it and if you want, I would love to help you to get there.

Do you want to lose 5, 8, 10, 15, 20 pounds? Easy, but please forget about any type of fitness program until you are about to reach your goal, then, you can establish your workout plan, but only then. I will explain you why.

what a feeling!

# REASONS FOR THIS BOOK : YOU

The title of this book could seem like a joke but the results will surprise you.

What I am proposing to you here is to ask yourself the same question that opened my eyes: WHY NOT ME?

This theory, as simple as it is, offers the tools to be a motivated person to take that decision and achieve the goal, your goal.

But this guide. this book is about YOU. You, having fun and enjoying what you do. You, knowing that you are free to choose your activities and to do with your life as you please. When you are doing what you really want to do, fun is always present. The goal will still be accomplished but in your own way, at the time that suits you best and always aligned to your own rhythm; no-one else's music, your tune.

For many people the process of losing weight seems like a burden that makes you feel, even before you start the diet-workout plan, depressed, sad, and your happiness is temporarily taking away, but you accept that as the price you pay to achieve the weight you want.

But in reality, these are just concepts and ideas that others make us believe.

If you read again the beginning of this page, you will realize that all that is just not true. Here I tell you again:

When you are doing what you really want to do, fun is always present. The goal will still be accomplished but in your own way, at the time that suits you best and always aligned to your own rhythm; no-one else's music, your tune.

I lost my weight easily and with pleasure, and saw results every day since the very first day. Why? Because I did it my way, and I certainly knew that if I would have combined my new way of eating with a workout routine, I will have quit the plan the second day!

Diet with exercise, does not work!!!!! I will explain why.

Time and time again life has shown us that easy does it. Life is really not that complicated! If you were to talk to a serene and contented older person you admire, and ask them where the source of such calmness and ease comes from, their answer would always be simple, easy, back to basics; easy living: easy food, easy fun, easy pace. They might have had a hard life without the technological advances we now enjoy, but their response to ills and troubles were often simple. Of course now life has developed and we want and should have more. *This book* shows you how to achieve what you want in a gentle, easy, fun way. This book is a simple and easy guide to a happier, more motivated, healthier, sexier and beautiful you.

It might seem a little nonsense right now, but how would you know if you haven't tried it? please remember that the idea is to always keep it simple and effective, the only goal now is to get in those jeans, the six pack will come later.

With this concept you can build your own way to lose weight, and you will decide when is the right moment to start exercising, but that is only if you want to exercise, meaning that to lose weight you don't have to run, jump, workout, in fact, that will only delay the process and will only make you tired and will motivate you to stop the diet (or your new way of eating).

When you have reached your goal and feel your success, you will naturally be a better, more contented person to be around. The fact that you feel good, you look good and you have reached the success you worked for, will transform you into the sexy woman you really are.

# MY STRATEGY

Owning a good pair of fitted and flattering pair of jeans is a must. Jeans don't lie, they are like good friends: comfortable, easy going, if treated right they can last a very long time and they always tell the truth. There is no hiding from your jeans. How do I manage to walk through my clean and organised house feeling good, looking great in my favourite pair of jeans and totally relaxed?

It sounds simple, but in reality for many people, a moment like this is not likely to happen very often. Do you often find yourself feeling uncomfortable, blotted and turning blue from lack of circulation because you are wearing your favourite pair of jeans? There is not bull shitting your jeans; they tell it like it is.

Following my simple life strategy, the first thing I do when I wake up in the morning is walk to the bathroom, turn the light on, get on the scale and check my weight but don't do it because I have to but because I like it. Without a body that I am happy to live and play with, life would be kind of boring. Do you know how much fun you can have with a body that's healthy, at the right weight and fit? You can have unlimited and sexy fun in the most unexpected ways! All that I write here is my truth, it's what works for me, but it might not be necessarily the truth for you. You will get the idea and can shift it around if you want to make it your own. Again, this is my truth but give it some consideration even if it sounds a world away of who you think you are, you might discover something about yourself. If I didn't take care of my body, my life would be incomplete. I am sure you have heard this expression many times before: how can I take care of others if I don't take care of myself first? Boring, but so true.

Looking after my body doesn't mean looking for a perfect body. It is all about my own body, my own shape, it doesn't have to look like someone else's body, it is me and my body just doing the best we can with what we have. It is about feeling sexy, happy and thankful for having this body. This body is all mine, nobody else can claim it, isn't that a wonderful fact? Are you happy and thankful for the body you have? Maybe not now, but you can change that.

Now back to my daily strategy. As I said before, I weigh myself everyday right after I get up. I know there are plenty of people out there telling us to weight ourselves just once a week or maybe don't weight ourselves at all! I have a problem with that. Look, how are you going to manage your weight if you don't check it? How can you manage anything without information? Isn't it easier to lose half of a pound than to lose one pound? How would you know that you need to lose that half of a pound before they get to be a pound if you haven't weighted yourself? You over indulge today and tomorrow you don't. Everything evens out easily, without struggle. I understand that there are women out there suffering from acute eating disorders that shouldn't weigh themselves at all and I also understand the theories some experts are trying to make us see, for example: what the scale shows could be water retention, or it could be that you are getting your period, or it could be that your muscles are getting bigger and stronger, it could be that you are a big boned kind of girl, but still healthy (I've never seen a big boned skeleton yet) and on and on they go. But how on earth do I know what's going on in my own body? How do I know if the weight comes from fat or from muscle? Am I bloated or just rosy cheeked and healthy? Am I over hydrated or dehydrated? Where can I find a straight answer? Better still, where can I find an answer that the experts agree on? I don't do any of this craziness anymore but honestly, in the past, as soon as I started to understand how to use the new best thing EVER to lose weight, when I just started to see a little light at the end of the tunnel, an expert of some sort wearing a white coat, would always come up and ruin it for me. He would appear out of the blue to inform me that the new best thing I just bought, that thing I poured all my hopes and soul (and money) into was actually a load of shit and potentially harmful to my health. What?? But don't despair, the expert would explain, here I have the real answer, the new real shit (sorry) the new real solution to all your body issues, but wait, there is more…

But, I just want to know how much I weigh! Do I really need to buy this sophisticated and very expensive piece of equipment that not only allows me the privilege to know my weight, but a lot of other things that I couldn't care less about: my fat percentage, my density of something, my hydration, my family history and a bunch of other stuff that I, in my humble opinion, DON'T WANT TO KNOW! I just want to know my weight today so I can compare it to my weight yesterday and see if I need to cut back a little bit TODAY to get back to where I was YESTERDAY. To me, it is that simple. I just want to know if yesterday's chocolate cake made a difference in my weight today and if it did, I can do something about it today, nothing harsh, no drastic diets, your weight doesn't need to get out of hand because you weighed yourself just yesterday, so cutting down here and there will do, maybe skip the cappuccino today and that will get you back to the weight you like in a day. When you weigh yourself on a daily basis, you get to know your own body very well, a lot better than using all those gadgets and percentages. You understand why your body is doing what it's doing, you know you are getting your period, you know that certain foods make you bloated, you know what types of food make you put on weight faster than other foods, you know where that little extra weight came from and you fix it today, not on your once a week weigh-in. Cut back today and the problem is fixed today, the easy way, back to basics. You will know your body well (after all it belongs to you, doesn't it?) you will understand your body's ups and downs, in other words you will be able to listen to what your body has been trying to tell you for years: when it comes to your body, you are the expert. Forget about all that nonsense and impracticality. To manage anything, including your weight, you need to be informed at all times so you can do something about it NOW, not next Friday. Simple.

So, back to the strategy. If, after I weigh myself in the morning, I find that my weight is the same as the day before or even a little less, I am in for a good start! The pleasure I feel walking to my closet with the freedom to pick any item of clothing I own, knowing that it will fit and it will look good, knowing that I will be comfortable for the rest of the day. All these small things give me an injection of energy and wellbeing that stretches throughout my day; helping me do all the things I need to do throughout the day with gusto!

Loving your body and taking care of yourself can bring you a sense of well being that prepares and motivates you to be productive and proactive in all areas of your life. Learning to love and cherish your own individual body is a tool you can always use to bring joy into your life whenever and wherever you want.

After checking my weight, I go to the kitchen and spoil myself with an exquisite cup of coffee.It might sound superficial to many, but to me this is the foundation for the rest of my day, because if I feel at ease in my own body and in my clothes, I am better prepared to focus on other things. I don't need to use my body as an excuse for neglecting the other things in my life. I don't need to obsess over my body; I don't need to say to myself: if only I could lose weight! Or if only I could have her body! No, my body is well looked after by me, it looks good and I am happy with it.

## Love your sexy body and make the most of it

If you are out in a public place and I were to ask you to have a good look around to point out the difference, if any, between women who love themselves and those who don't, would you be able to do it?

If you pay attention, you will. In fact, it is not difficult to distinguish one from the other. A woman who loves herself has a different posture than one who doesn't. She stands tall and walks with some dignity and plenty of confidence; you somehow get the sense that she enjoys who she is. It is not only about how she looks, it is something else that she transmits to others; something that can't be pinpointed but that certainly attracts people, almost like a magnetic field where people can't help but turn around and look.

She would look groomed and well dressed and normally she wouldn't be in a hurry. But, you may ask, what has being in a hurry to do with any of this? A woman who cares about herself will give priority to her well being. She does things faster because she is effective and very practical, but she does them without agitation and she knows when to stop to avoid feeling stressed out.

Look, let me be frank, it doesn't matter who you are or what you do, how old you are or how much you weigh; you know (don't deny it, no one can hear you) that getting attention for the right reasons feels very good, very sexy. It boosts your energy and your confidence, you want to eat the right foods and you want to be kind to your body because you know you are hot and you want that HOTNESS to last as long as possible. This is sexy.

Don't hide your body with layers and layers of fabric, not only are layers unsexy, but also extremely unflattering. They make you look bigger and draw attention to the very thing you are trying to hide. They make you look (and feel) like a circus tent, so don't be surprised if children (not men) follow you around. We'll study this point in detail in the Dress Skinny Rule.

If you are lucky enough to have big boobs or a shapely bottom or any other type of curves in your magnificent body, ENJOY them and let others enjoy them too by SHOWING them in all their sexy glory. Keep in mind that all this showing must be done in an elegant, chic (not cheap) way. Learning to show off your body is an art in itself. Accentuate, draw attention to the parts of your body that you love and are proud of and the bits of your body you are not too crazy about won't get a glance; all eyes will be glued to those spectacular boobs, butt or any other part of your womanly shape.

WARNING: It is very important that you don't confuse curves and shapes with fat and flabby. A lot of women tend to do that and, truth be told, it is not pleasant on the eye and a little bit rude. If you have a big tummy, you don't need to wear the above mentioned circus tent, BUT please don't wear that cute little tank top either. It is not sexy at all.

If we love and take care of what really matters - our health and our bodies, everything else will fall into place. We should spoil and be kind to our bodies at every opportunity we get and as often as we can. Your body will respond to your attention. Think about your body as your very own fountain of fun and enjoyment. Your body is grateful and very forgiving and will always react to your kindness and care by looking great and feeling even better!

Every once in a while try lying down with your legs up, close your eyes and let your body rest and recharge itself, you will instantly feel better.

Love your skin and love your hands and feet. Eat well and try to sleep enough; you will get it all back.

You earned it.

I will let you have a peek into some of my sexy diet tips later on in this guide; you'll be surprise in what I have to tell you.

## Dress Skinny

*"I love big challenges and small dresses"...*

How on earth can I dress skinny when I am fat? I hear you, do not despair. This question is what makes this rule one of the most important of all the sexy rules, dress skinny!

How can you eat and enjoy food and never feel like you are on a diet? I do it every day, constantly. I love food, I eat all the time, but I have discovered the secret to staying thin, Dress Skinny.

Many women give permission to their bodies to be fat, sorry to be so blunt but yes that is the truth. I am not talking about the many women that are suffering with serious eating disorders. I am talking about the average women out there, the ones that lose 2 pounds and gain back 3, the ones that enjoy eating and don't want to miss out, the ones with the constant battle with the scales. You? Maybe?

Giving permission to your body to get fat is very easy to do, the only thing you need to do is to open your closet door, reach for the biggest item of clothing you own (a big summer dress, big trousers, big leggings, x-large t-shirts, long flowing and layered skirts, you name it) put them on and try to convince others and especially YOURSELF that you like COMFORT, what's wrong with that? That's the type of girl you are! You have no need to show bits and pieces of your flesh because you are all about COMFORT and being down to earth, you have errands to do, kids to pick up; why do I need to wear those skinny jeans? I'll tell you why, but I warn you it won't be COMFORTABLE to read it. The extra large items you are wearing together with those words you are trying to believe in are the best and fastest way to achieve: Disaster! Once you are inside those big clothes, you have given your body and your mind permission to overeat.

Dressing big gives you more room for food. When you are wearing big loose clothes, you don't know (and sometimes pretend not to know) if you have eaten too much, you don't feel the pain. When you are wearing tight fitted clothes, you are able to notice if you have had enough, you can't ignore it; the discomfort will be there to remind you and it will stay there until you either change your clothes and put something COMFORTABLE on or until you stop eating. That is up to you, to go home (so you can continue eating as much as you like and remain comfortable) and miss all the fun or stay put and enjoy the moment, relaxed and happy knowing that you made the right decision: you are there to have fun, to share time (not food) with friends, to enjoy the moment, you were NOT invited to that lovely gathering to stuff your face with food. Sounds harsh but sometimes we need to hear the truth.

What I really want to say to you here is simple: The problem is not what you eat but the amount that you eat. I eat everything. I am relaxed when I eat. I know the clothes I chose to wear this morning will let me know when I have had enough. What are you choosing to wear today?

When you dress skinny you stay skinny; if you are not thin you will immediately look thinner and you will like that feeling so much that there is no going back to the extra large COMFORTABLE clothes.

When you dress skinny, all your womanly curves and your sexy shape and form, pops up. There is nothing sexier...

## Take a risk, comfort zone means boring

Dare yourself to do that very thing, that one thing that not long ago you would have never even considered doing! It's just NOT you, not sensible enough! And, may I ask, for what purpose? Where is the logic behind it? Have you lost your mind? Am I crazy? Mmm...

I don't think I can completely express in words the pleasure, the high you feel after you have achieved the goals you set out to get. To take that project all the way to the end, to face your fears and push them out of the way and take a risk. To do that one thing you thought impossible. Trust me when I tell you, it is one of the best experiences of your entire life. Don't miss it if you can, there is so much to learn from it that will transform your life and the way you look at things. You will want more and you will know that you can get more. What a lesson to teach and share around: You lived a life where fear was ignored and it just wasn't an option.

So, please listen to me because I am about to give you another one of my tips: GET YOUR BUTT OUT THERE AND DO IT! You sexy thing...

# MY SEXY DIET TIPS

## Gym Owners, Personal Trainers and Diet Specialists:

Please be aware, the contents of this chapter may offend you. Understand that what I mention in this chapter are just tips, diet tips; we women do it all the time, we like helping each other out. This is not personal. This is not a lifestyle change. Exercise is good for you, my sexy readers know that, my women friends know it too, we all do: Exercise is good for you. Now take a deep breath and let your sexy, rock-solid six pack abs relax... that's better, now go for a run Champion!

## I DON'T EXERCISE WHEN I WANT TO LOSE WEIGHT

I am not a doctor, so please don't assume that I know what's right. I know what is right for me, but I don't know if it is good for you. These are just little tips that work for me. Be sensible and practical, and always talk to your doctor.

My number one tip for keeping a slim, sexy body is this:

When I want to lose weight, I don't exercise much at the beginning of my diet programme. Actually, I don't exercise at all for a while. I know this is the complete opposite of what the experts tell us, but it makes sense and works for me.

When you are taking your first steps towards a slimmer, sexier body, your body reacts. Days, weeks, months or maybe even years of eating carbs and sugars of all types and to suddenly stop, just like that, will get your body a little confused (to say the least). It is going to be hard for both your body and your mind. You start detoxifying, you feel hungry, deprived and lonely. There is nothing sexy about it. You feel like crap, but you are determined to see the body you know is hidden under there.

Instead of treating yourself a bit nicer for being such a trooper, instead of quietly going through this process in a dignified way until you see some results, instead of giving yourself a hug and having a little cry, instead of giving yourself all the extra care you know you need while you go through this fragile but crucial stage in the programme, instead of all that care, you are told to: GET OUT THERE AND MOVE IT! Are you kidding me? Why? Aren't you suffering enough already? You are confused and tired from the lack of your daily sugar intake and you are told to move it? Sweat it out? Are you mad?

And of course there you go, like the good girl you are, because this time you are going to do it! This is it!! You sign up for one, or more, of the following options found in the gym: A) Pumping iron so heavy that your risk of getting a hernia or haemorrhoids increases dramatically B) Doing RPM - this is cycling in a small and dark room with disco lights and very LOUD music that won't let you hear whatever it is the instructor is shouting at you C) You sign up for a Step Class - get on and off this silly little step placed in front of you while following a very complicated dance routine that would be better suited in the movie FAME; the list is endless, so many options to get you in shape and most of them just plain mean and embarrassing. And what's the story with the mirrors? Are they getting them for free? The bloody things are everywhere! Do they think you enjoy watching yourself jumping up and down while looking fat and uncoordinated? BUT, this time it's going to work! You have had enough of all this fat!! So, there you are, sweating (not perspiring but sweating, like a pig), uncomfortable and out of breath. All this effort and indignity only to find, when you get home that you are hungrier than ever before. You are exhausted, hungry, detoxifying, miserable and still FAT! And you wonder why you quit. Please! When you are consuming the amount of calories you need to lose those pounds, you are hungry. You are hungry at least until your stomach shrinks a little and your body has settled. Isn't it absurd that to complete the whole drama you have to hit the streets and go for a run?

Being hungry, grumpy, deprived, humiliated and tired doesn't do it for me. This combination is too much and too complicated for my liking, it stresses me out so I don't do it.

Let's bring some sexy practicality back to our lives. After years of trying, I now know that I cannot start my diet programme and exercise routine at exactly the same time. Some people can and love it, but I can't and hate it. It just doesn't work for me so I don't do it.

Here is what works for me, my Sexy Diet Tip 1:

There are two stages in my Getting Back into Shape routine:

1. - Reach your target weight or at least get closer in numbers to the weight you want.
2. - Tone those muscles: GET OUT THERE AND MOVE IT! Yes, bring it on baby! Now, I can handle it.

Another thing I DON'T and NEVER will do, is to try to lose weight by exercising only. It does not work. Listen, you can have a dance off with your aerobics instructor and win, but if you keep eating the same way it won't work. Yes, you will get muscles but you won't see them until you stop overeating, and the reason for that is simple, those muscles you are working so hard to get, are hidden under all the fat that you are carrying. You will not only look bigger but you will look kind of masculine? I don't think that's the look you are after, unless you are planning to join the Marines.

I lost 10 pounds while standing like a mummy from some ancient civilization, so still was I that even my child checked my breathing every once in a while. I concentrated on just one thing, to get my eating under control. I stayed put and lost the weight. Then and only then I started moving, first like a toddler learning to walk, until I was ready to go back to the gym and tone those muscles! Back in shape and looking great my way, in a comfortable, elegant and sexy way.

Why don't you allow your body to lose those pounds in a serene and relaxed way? Then, when you are ready, when you are not so hungry anymore, when your sugar levels are more balanced, THEN slowly you can start training to tone those muscles but in a practical way, without desperation because your clothes already fit you. Does that make sense? That is what I do, and for me it works. Go ahead and go for a walk, get some fresh air, it can only do you good but don't overdo anything. You need the strength to keep you focused on your diet plan. Your body will tell you when it is time to exercise and tone so you go to the gym, simple. Don't try to run before you master your walking, you will only fall and hurt yourself.

Experiment both ways and see which one works for you. If dieting and exercising at the same time is making you miserable, stop and do it in stages, in a more practical way. Listen to your body a bit more. Start cutting down the calories and wait until all those horrible first few days are gone, allow your body to settle and comfortably ease into your new, healthier and sexier eating habits. Those first few pounds always go away quite easily at the beginning and that is encouraging, so you start weighing yourself, you start learning how your body works and with this information you are ready to manage your body and your weight better forever.

When I start eating healthier and less, my body is happy. The food I eat when trying to lose weight is delicious but simple and not too much of it. I don't let myself get too hungry, because being too hungry doesn't work for me. I have a snack if I need it and keep going.

You will notice that when you start losing weight in a gentler way, you start feeling more comfortable with your body and you want to keep going because you like that feeling. After a while, not only will you feel comfortable with your body but you will actually start liking it; your body will feel good to you. You will want to keep this process going because maybe, for the first time in your life, you and your body are becoming friends instead of enemies. You will discover an appreciation for the gift that is your body and who knows? You might end up actually loving it and wanting to protect it better.

To me, this is sexy, effective and gentle practicality at its best.

Sexy Diet Tip 2:

I eat and drink what I want but in small quantities and with a strategy. Keep in mind that dieting without a strategy will not work. This is my strategy: when I want something sweet, an apple won't do the trick. When I have a craving for something sweet I eat something sweet, because if I don't, I feel deprived and think about that something sweet all day long. So, I have a small piece of chocolate or a little cookie, only once a day (that is enough, once a day. You really must stop all that craving, all the time; you are not pregnant, you just want to eat).

If I am hungry in between meals I have a piece of fruit or a cup of yogurt mixed with pieces of apple or I have a skinny cappuccino with a low calorie cracker.

I don't over eat or under eat. I don't eat a whole bar of chocolate or a packet of cookies. I would feel uncomfortable and moody if I did that. If I eat too much in between meals, it kills the pleasure of my next meal. I feel bloated and that wonderful feeling you get when you start losing weight and getting in shape goes away. To me it's not worth it, especially after you survived those first few days of hell at the start of your diet.

Sexy Diet Tip 3:

This is what I normally eat when trying to lose a few pounds. Again, it works for me, I don't know if it will work for you. If you like it and it works for you, great! But if it doesn't, you must find what works best for you.

Breakfast:

A big cup of coffee with skinny milk and a little sugar or stevia (a natural sweetener)
2 low fat (and huge) crispbreads (around 16 calories each and very filling) or
1 piece of toast
1 egg or some cheese on top of my bread or cracker (it doesn't matter what kind of cheese but aim for the low fat variety if you can, Edam is always a lighter choice, up to you). If you want to eat something hot in the morning, put the cheese on top of the crispbread and microwave for 50 seconds until it melts, delicious!
Please note: when I say SOME cheese I don't mean ALL the cheese, no little layers and layers of cheese on top of your crispbread please, it is not a Mexican taco, aim for 1 or 2 thin layers, always handle cheese with a lot of caution.

Mid morning:
Another cup of coffee
A mandarin or an apple
If I'm still hungry I have 1 or 2 crispbreads with a little cheese or ham.

Lunch:

Soup: homemade, in a tin or instant (whatever suits me at the moment). Try broccoli soup, it's good for you and delicious. You can find very healthy and low calorie soups in the supermarket or make your own, it is easy and you can make a big bowl and freeze it for later use.

To my soup I add huge amounts of vegetables (carrots, broccoli, peppers etc) until it is quite thick, then sprinkle some parmesan cheese on top and mix. I'll have the soup with 2 big crispbreads.

A glass of orange juice made from the juice of just one orange.

Mid Afternoon:

Coffee or tea

Some fruit

A cookie or a little piece of dark chocolate

Dinner:

A salad made of rucola or any other type of lettuce, tomatoes, peppers, olive oil, balsamic vinegar, cucumber and as many other vegetables I want. I season it with paprika.

I add some chicken, meat or fish. (Whatever is handy and easy)

I eat as much as I want from this salad.
If you want a hot meal stir fry the vegetables in a little oil and add the meat.
One corn tortilla or a pita bread ( put it in the sandwich toaster for 4 minutes)

Dessert:
Soya chocolate pudding (low fat)
Cup of coffee (I drink cappuccino with two little spoons of sugar)

That's it. It couldn't get any easier.

## Other sexy diet tips

I don't eat too many fruits when dieting because I either put on weight or don't lose any. I eat all the vegetables I want, but I am careful with fruits, I try to stick to oranges, mandarins, pears and apples. I try not to eat bananas, grapes or watermelon.

Again, this is true for me but maybe not for you, weigh yourself and try different fruits to see how your body reacts; remember it is all about what your body is telling you.

I don't eat starches like potatoes, rice or pasta unless I am eating out.

I eat very little bread, sometimes a slice for breakfast if my weight is ok that morning or if I feel hungry. Wholemeal bread (not white) is always best.

Finally one of my best sexy slimming tips:

Think skinny and dress skinny. As we discussed on the Dress Skinny Chapter, if you dress big your body relaxes and expands making it easier to overeat.

Keep talking and listening to your body, it does what you want and is very grateful.

Keep telling yourself that your body is trim and fit until you get it, the power of the mind is amazing, believe me,it works.

And ...


Let's keep the simple and the sexy going, just follow these simple but wise rules:

Eat well to be, to feel and to look great.

Feel sexy, think sexy, talk sexy and BE sexy no matter what.

Never stop looking for passion in everything you do from this moment on.

All the best...


Theira  Añez &  Delia Añez authors of  "me, Me,ME Oops@ why not? And "The 10 sexy rules"

 Theira Añez: Author of "Cadenas Invisibles"